Breath Therapy

For

Long Covid

Dermot Ryan B.A.

CONTENTS

<u>Covid-19 Recovery Breathing Therapy</u>

1. Introduction

You are interested in this topic because you have contracted Covid-19. You could either be in the early phases of it, you could have had it for a little while or you may already be on the mend. It is very likely that you are experiencing breathing difficulties, a drop in your blood oxygen levels, perhaps damage to the lungs and on top of this the uncertainty that Covid-19 brings. You are probably experiencing higher levels of anxiety, stress and even depression.

Recovery begins by focusing on your breath. The better shape your lungs are in, the better of you are going to feel. Of course, you will have more energy and then you can counter one of the main problems with Covid-19, which is a drop in blood oxygen levels. To assist you on your journey to recovery, I have put together four very accessible breathing practices. These simple techniques can be used to help address many of the negative states that are brought on by Covid-19. These practices are to be used over a 14-day period, twice a day, morning, and evening and on an empty stomach. It is also preferable to wear loose fitting clothing, so that the body does not have a feeling of being restricted in any way.

They are:

1. Deep Breathing – Learning how to Breathe
2. Kapalbhati – Shining Skull Breath
3. Brahamari – Black Bee Breath – Humming
4. Rhythmic Breathing for Health and Wellbeing

2. Corona Virus and your Lungs

How does Corina Virus – Covid-19 affect the lungs?

Covid-19 kills us by attacking the lungs and making our breathing difficult. You can think of the lungs a bit like an upside-down tree. The trunk is your windpipe, and the branches are the bronchi of the lungs. These bronchi get smaller and smaller like branches until they end in tiny air sacks called alveoli. In healthy lungs the oxygen crosses the alveoli into the blood vessels and from there, oxygen is transported to the rest of your body. With covid-19, as the virus replicates, it causes your own immune system to go into hyper drive. White blood cells trigger the inflammation response which in turn rallies more immune systems cells to kill infected cells. The fallout from this ongoing battle between your immune system and the virus leaves behind pus. This is made up of excess fluid and dead cells which line the walls of the alveoli. The thicker that this wall gets, the harder it is to transfer the oxygen that you breath in, into your blood. This results in respiratory tract symptoms such as coughing, fever and shortness of breath. This can also lead to Hypoxia which can in turn lead to multiple organ damage through oxygen deprivation.

This results in a feeling of being short on breath, but many people will also have low oxygen levels and not even be aware that this is happening. Testing oxygen levels using an oximeter has become quite popular. Normal blood oxygen levels are around 95% to 100% and indicate that the lungs are functioning properly. With Covid-19, blood oxygen saturation can get as low as 50%. This plummeting oxygen level can cause further damage to organs including the lungs, the heart, liver, kidneys, and the brain and in extreme cases leads to death. Therefore, it is important to use the main tool we have which is, breathing, to be able to improve blood oxygen levels. We can use proper, controlled and targeted breathing to clear out the phlegm build-up inside the lungs and to reduce chronic inflammation. This is exactly what the techniques in this short book can do for you. When putting the techniques into practice, you will find that a lot of the anxiety and negative feelings caused by exposure to Covid-19 will also be eased, and a state of control can return once again.

As you progress through this course, you will learn to breathe deeply and consciously. Over the two weeks recommended, you will gradually, step by step, feel the healing results that conscious breathing will bring to you. Make sure that you rest when you need to and take it at your own pace. If the breathing practices happen to start a cough and bring up phlegm etc., let it, and then resume the practice when you can. You may find that these breathing practices are the foundation for a future practice. Conscious breathing and Breathwork are much more than simply fixing what is wrong but can also be used as a starting point to discover many more layers of insight into your mind, body, and self.

 If during this course you would like to reach out any time with questions, I look forward to hearing from you at dryanyoga@gmail.com

3. Good Posture for Breathing

Let us look for a moment about how you want to position your body to attain the maximum benefit from your breathing. We will then follow this by re-learning how to breathe, something you may have thought you were doing correctly all along.

For body position there will be three choices: Firstly, you can sit on a solid chair, or cross-legged on the floor. For this position, just be aware that your spine should be as straight as is comfortable for you, and should not be supported i.e., your back should not be touching the back of the chair. If sitting on a solid chair, both feet should be flat on the floor. If you imagine pushing your lower back in towards your navel, this can help to avoid the back and shoulder from rounding.

For your second position, you may lay down on your back on the floor, feet, and legs apart, and hands and arms away from the body, your palms facing up towards the ceiling.

Finally, laying down on your belly on the floor, preferably on a yoga/exercise mat as you do not want any dust particles entering your nasal passage and lungs. Let your big toes touch each other and let your ankles relax and move outwards. Place one hand on top of the other and rest your forehead on the back of your upper hand. This prone position, known as Crocodile Pose in Yoga, has been found to be the most effective position to increase oxygen levels in Covid-19 patients.

It is very important that no matter which position you choose; you are comfortable and warm. Use cushions, blankets and whatever makes these positions as comfortable and cosy as possible. Also, try and make sure that there are no nagging pains in your joints or muscles, so that you can give one hundred percent attention to the exercises. Of course, you can mix and match these positions throughout the two-week programme.

To finish, you may need to adjust your shoulders. From long term bad habit, we tend to lift our shoulders up towards our ears and bring our shoulders closer together, creating tension in our upper body and putting strain on our upper lungs. To ease this tension, try to push your shoulders away from each other and at the same time let them drop down. Extend your neck by slowly moving it back and forth and try to get the feeling of it extending upwards with each movement.

4. Shut Your Mouth

Is a simple thing like letting air in and out of your mouth and down into your lungs creating a you that is no longer functioning to your full health potential? The answer is a resounding Yes. Read any writings by renowned Buteko breathing specialist, Patrick McKeown or even the short experiment by James Nestor in his recent book, "Breath".

Why are these habits bad for your health? Why do you need to learn to do something that you have been doing since birth and that you do without thinking every minute of every day? You started your life as the perfect breather and despite what we think, when babies are not crying, they have their mouths shut and are breathing in and out through their nostrils. As we grow up, we unlearn this and slowly our heavy jaw begins to drop. We start breathing mostly through or mouths. We have become the only animals on the planet that mouth breathe.

If we are not doing this, we are, what is termed "gymnastic" breathing. We are expanding our chest when inhaling and contracting our chest when exhaling. We pull our abdomen in when we inhale and relax our abdomen when we exhale.

A further habit we tend to develop is vertical breathing. This is the habit of letting our shoulders rise on an inhale and drop down when exhaling.

These three most common breathing habits are having a detrimental effect on our health and I could go as far as to say, killing us. It is hard to believe that breathing can kill you. Let me be a little less dramatic. Breathing incorrectly is "slowly" killing you. It is also increasing your dental bills. It is stopping you controlling your weight. It is giving you asthma and reducing your lung capacity. This, in addition to Covid-19 and your ability to recover is a deadly cocktail.

Along with giving you lower back pain, it is increasing damaging issues with your neck and shoulders. It is increasing your risk of having cardiac and lung problems. It is affecting your ability to control your weight. It is giving you sleepless nights. It is damaging your health in these and many other ways, but most importantly it is reducing your chances of making a full recovery from the effects of Covid-19.

The art of un-learning these bad breathing habits is one of the most easily accessible health remedies available. The three words, **Shut Your Mouth**, will save you endless problems. Get into the habit of repeating this mantra to yourself throughout your day. It will help you unlearn bad habits. It will be your first guide on the road of new breathing techniques.

5. Diaphragm Strengthening

At this point I would like to mention that there are certain things that you can do to build up the strength of your diaphragm, the primary breathing muscle. First and foremost, anytime that you put a restriction on the air flow into your lungs, it makes your diaphragm work a bit harder as it pulls the air deeper into your body. It also helps to lower high blood pressure, improve brain function, and improves the transfer of oxygen throughout the body.

Of course, as we have seen, breathing through your nose because the nose is again a smaller passageway than the mouth, restricts the flow of air and so strengthens the Diaphragm. Of course, focusing on this throughout your daily life while walking, running, sleeping and particularly during the breathing practices in this course are all going to be done through the nose and we will slowly build the strength of the diaphragm.

Another technique to help with the strengthening of the diaphragm is called Ujjayi breathing, also called Ocean breathing. I am mentioning this breathing exercise now, but it should only be used when you have already completed this two-week course and your diaphragm has begun to strengthen at a slow and steady pace. I find that this very simple breathing technique really helps me to focus inwardly and shut out peripheral noise and sound in my immediate surroundings. It helps focus the mind on the breath and builds an awareness of the health of my breathing in the moment. Sometimes it sounds like cars on a wet road, the wind passing through trees and even Darth Vader. It gives us the opportunity to judge the quality and smoothness of the breath and the progress we have made.

Simply put, we are constricting the flow of breath in our throat on both the inhale and the exhale. Of course, we are sitting in a comfortable position, with our spines straight and body relaxed. Our mouth is closed, and we are only breathing through our nostrils. Initially it may help to let your chin slightly drop towards your chest to get the feeling and sound of restricted breath, but once attained, lift the chin up, parallel to the floor. Even though the breath is slightly restricted, it should still flow softly and evenly on both the inhale and the exhale. The sound is the key to this soft, even, effortless, subtle, and so on.

In the beginning you will probably find that exhaling is easier than inhaling because when you inhale again you are having to resist against that smaller aperture. This is perfectly normal, but with practice, your aim is to make the inhale and exhale both equal length and equal sound.

6. Stretch Your Body

It can be of great benefit to do some easy body stretches before focussing on the practice of breathing. We hold tension in our bodies whether physical or emotional. You may have been hospitalised or have been bed-ridden for some time, so there may be some degeneration of your muscle mass and strength. If we mentally scan our bodies, we can get a feel for places where these weaknesses and tensions are lodged. I always tell my students that the first place to check is the jaw and then move slowly around the body from there, mentally releasing tension as they move through the body, right down to the toes. Whether sitting, lying down, or standing, move your body into positions that are not usual for you. There is no need for a standard set of motions or poses for this practice. Maybe bend forward and try to touch your toes. Swing your arms slowly around your body. Lift your arms above your head. Look over your shoulders. Look at the floor and then maybe look slowly up to the ceiling. Use your exhalations to release any tension and picture your inhalations bringing new energy and strength into your body. Building up your imagination can be very effective too.

7. Learning to Breath

You have kept yourself alive for all these years, so you should really be an expert at breathing. Like everything else we do, we can fall into bad habits, so let us suspend all we think we know and begin. For the purposes of this exercise, we will use a hard chair to sit on.

Sit upright, out at the edge of your seat, so that your spine is not being supported. Try to picture your spine as a straight line from the chair all the way up to the base of your skull. Close your mouth! You only inhale and exhale through your nostrils…. take a deep breath in …and exhale….and again….and again…. You will notice that when you do this, you slightly rise up when you inhale and move down when you exhale…Perfect? Well, it is not perfect, at all.

Now, place your hands on your sides, your index fingers tucked slightly beneath your lowest rib. When you inhale, feel your elbows move away from your body. Now do this a few times…. lovely…. now keep your hands there, and we will do some more inhales and exhales, but when you inhale now, first, push your navel towards the wall in front of you, then let your elbows push out and then fill the upper part of your lungs and finally let the breath fill your throat. This is the three parts of correct breathing. If you like to add another layer, it might be nice to add another layer when beginning. So, four stages…belly, elbows, upper lungs, throat and then a nice long exhale. This may be very new to you and after many years of vertical breathing. It may feel strange and it is easy to slip back to habits shaped by many years of unconscious breathing habits. Stick with it and retrain your body and mind.

Now let us focus on the exhale. When you exhale, slowly let the air leave your throat, then your lungs and finally your belly. Pull your bellybutton/navel back in towards your spine, trying to push all the air out from the bottom of your lungs. Practice at a slow pace and do not put any stress into the action. Just do what is 100% comfortable and steady. Always try to make sure that your exhalation is longer than your inhalation...it is the exhalation that reduces your heart rate and your blood pressure...the optimum is that your exhalation is twice the length of your inhalation, but this comes with a lot of practice and concentration...This is correct breathing, and it is probably a lot different from what you have been doing for all your life. When I initially asked you to Inhale and Exhale, you were vertical breathing. Up and down, but you did not always do this. When you were born and for the first few years of your life, you breathed correctly, but then you became self-aware, you were told to stand tall, tuck in your tummy, have presence and this led you down the path of vertical or gymnastic breathing. This vertical motion places a lot of stress on your shoulders and neck. We spend a lot of our time on computers and other devices, leading to a myriad of neck and shoulder issues that are having an increasing negative impact on our health. If we repeat an incorrect motion 23,000 per day, every day, then the consequences can be easily identified.

For the purposes of this programme and for your future, this is the way you should be breathing from now on. You will find yourself drifting back to your old habits, but with practice and attention, these lapses will become less and less frequent.

8. Kapalabhati – Pump Action Breathing – Shining Skull

While generally regarded as a cleansing exercise in Yoga, Kapalabhati is an ideal practice to prepare the body and lungs for an extended breathing practice. It is important to do this breathing exercise at the beginning of your routine and it is also important that you do this practice in a very gentle way. This practice is not recommended during pregnancy or for those with hypertension or panic disorder. The alternative practice in this case is Ujjayi Breath, which we discussed earlier.

To begin, as we always do, get into the most comfortable position of your choice. Begin to relax by breathing deep and long, extending your exhalations to increase the relaxation messages to the body and mind. This initiates your parasympathetic nervous system and messages the body to "rest and digest". Maybe you can start by inhaling for a slow count of three and exhaling for a slow count of four and throughout your two weeks programme, extend this to four/five and then to four/six. Never put your body, mind, or lungs under any stress. This is not a competition.

When ready, inhale to 70/80% of your lung capacity, pause, and then exhale through the nose forcefully, as if you are sneezing. You will feel your abdomen engaging and your navel moving towards your spine. Repeat a few times to help your body get used to the feeling. You may feel a little lightheaded, but this is normal and nothing to worry about.

When you are ready, start your practice with 10 forceful exhalations through the nostrils, and then slowly exhale completely. Each cycle should be one second and the tempo should be even. Inhale deeply and exhale completely twice and on the 3rd inhale, hold your breath. Close your eyes and focus on the area between your eyebrows or the area at your heart centre. Hold your breath for as long as you are comfortable. Again, always keeping in mind that your lungs should never be under any stress. If your breath hold is five seconds, then accept that. Over your fourteen days, this will slowly improve, but the key to progress is "slow and steady". Remember there is no benefit to holding your breath for an extended period if it stresses the lungs and body. If there is any breathlessness, then the breath has been held for too long.

Now, repeat the process two more times, the second time with 12 exhalations and the third time with 15 exhalations. Over time, and when you are fully recovered, you can advance your practice and increase the forceful exhalations, always keeping in mind that the most benefit from this exercise is attained by working within your capacity and never being breathless. Try not to put the cart before the horse.

What is the Science?

During the practice of Kapalabhatti, the levels of Carbon Dioxide (CO_2) in the blood substantially drop quickly.

Although this is abnormal, it is beneficial to the body. It is especially beneficial for those suffering from Long Covid, because, as we mentioned earlier, the levels of Oxygen (O2) in the body drop from Covid-19 infection. The normal level of CO2 is re-established soon after the end of the practice. So, what is the actual benefit of this practice and why do we do it to begin our therapy?

This temporary drop in CO2 in the blood give the cells a chance to eliminate their own CO2. As this happens, the cells become saturated with Oxygen and this activity is very important for those who are in recovery from this virus. It is also beneficial to the general population who live a mostly sedentary life. This cellular respiration harvests energy in the body for immediate or later use.

Along with purifying the lungs, increasing, and maintaining suppleness, the exercise builds and maintains the mobility of the diaphragm while strengthening the abdominal muscles.

Along with all this, it is a tonic for the whole nervous system. After the stress and fatigue dealing with Covid-19 , it is the ideal practice to recover lost vitality. Use it to regain freshness, clear the mind of that muddled feeling and banish any hint of lethargy and listlessness. Watch how regular practice will help you with your concentration levels and improves your memory.

9. Bhramari – Humming – Black Bee Breathing

Before we begin with this technique of breathing and humming, it is good that you have a little understanding and how this technique works. It helps to have practical evidence, so that you can have the faith to pursue the practice. When you know what is happening inside your body then it becomes easier to pursue the practice over the recommended fourteen days and hopefully making Breathwork part of your ongoing health regime.

When you eat food that is high in Nitrates, this is converted to Nitric Oxide in the body. These foods include Celery, Beetroot, Spinach and Lettuce. A recent study by the University of Exeter found that athletes who drank beetroot juice (480ml/1 Pint per day for 7 days) showed a huge reduction in the amount of oxygen required to perform exercise. The numbers were impressive with a 16% increase in endurance for cyclists. Coupled with a reduction in blood pressure, they concluded that this reduction in the need for oxygen to increase endurance could not be achieved by any other training method.

Nitric Oxide is a molecule that is produced naturally by your body. It is important for many aspects of your health. Its most important function is to relax the inner muscles of the blood vessels, causing them to widen and increase circulation. This is called vasodilation.

Nitric oxide production is essential for overall health because it allows blood, nutrients, and oxygen to travel to every part of your body effectively and efficiently. Most importantly for us, Nitric Oxide increases oxygen transfer in the lungs which is something that is lacking when we get sick with Coronavirus/Covid-19. Its other main function is that it serves as a host defence i.e., it protects the body from invasions by viruses, pathogens, bacteria etc. When they come in through the respiratory tract, they do not survive the presence of Nitric Oxide. Its function that is most pertinent to us is that it keeps the upper airways relatively sterile while transferring Oxygen more efficiently to our lungs.

Fortunately, there are many ways to maintain optimal levels of nitric oxide in your body. The most effective method is nasal breathing and to boost production exponentially, just hum while inhaling and exhaling through your nose. For the purposes of this two-week programme, we will only be using this technique while exhaling. Please note that Nitric Oxide is not produced when we breathe through our mouth, so this re-affirms the importance of nasal breathing. It is also interesting to note that in a Swedish

Study, it was found that Humming increased the production of NO, 15 to 20 times in the nasal passage and sinuses.

A word of warning - avoid mouthwash. Mouthwash kills many types of bacteria including the ones that produce nitric oxide. This limits the ability of your body to produce Nitric Oxide.

So, let us move on with the practice.

Sitting or lying in your chosen position, straight spine, inhale, and exhale deeply through the nose a few times. For us, the exhalation is of greater significance in this practice. When you are ready begin.

Inhale deeply and slowly begin to exhale. Slightly restrict the breath between the throat and the nasal passage. If you need to tuck your chin towards your chest to do this, that is perfectly fine. The best way to describe the sound is Ng. Let the sound become steady and even, no jumpiness or highs or lows. Exhale as slowly as you can without putting any pressure on your body or mind. Remove all the breath from your lungs by slowly letting your navel move towards your spine. Do not strain to make the sound last. It should fade away as if the bee is fading out of earshot, not stopping, just fading. This is an ideal practice to time, and it is generally recommended to do 3-5 minutes. Of course, it can also be done with several breaths, 5/7/10 etc. Take two to three long inhalations and exhalations between each practice. For such a simple calm practice, the physical benefits are enormous.

To begin, the sound of the exhalation may be a little jumpy with slight gaps, but this will improve and become continuous and unbroken.

The benefits of Brahmari are listed as:

- It increases the production on Nitric Oxide in the nasal passage
- It assists in the reduction of stress. ...

- It lowers blood pressure, thus relieving hypertension.
- It releases cerebral tension.
- It soothes the nerves.
- It stimulates the pineal and pituitary glands, thus supporting their proper functioning.
- It dissipates anger.
- It is helpful in preventing heart blockages
- It helps with inducing deep sleep

10. Breathing Rhythmically

For our final practice we are going to be practicing what is also known as Resonant Frequency Breathing. It is also called Coherent Breathing. This type of breathing has been tried and tested and has a multitude of very positive effects, both physically and mentally. It is a also a very simple practice and even though it is part of our recovery programme, it can be easily practiced throughout your day.

The basic idea of the practice is that you will be inhaling for six seconds and exhaling for six seconds. This will be practiced continuously, without pause – breathe in, breathe out. That is all you do and there is something that happens when you breath in this Rhythm. Of course, in the beginning you may not have the capacity for six inhales and exhales. Start with what feels good for you, even if it is 3/4/5, but keep the same rhythm for the inhale and the exhale. Over the two weeks you will easily get to six.

When you do get to six inhales and exhales, this will work out to be five breaths per minute. In your normal daily life you will breathe 12-15 times per minute. Physiologists have produced many papers on this rhythm of breathing. In a nutshell the overall effect is that your breath, your heart rate, and your blood pressure all begin to synchronize together. As the breathing slips into this mode the heart rate starts to speed up and slowdown in perfect synchronized relationship with the breath and on the other side of that the blood pressure starts to oscillate between high and low pressure in perfect timing with the heart and a perfect timing with the breath.

For those who have experienced Covid-19 and particularly where people do not get enough of blood oxygen pumping through the body, Resonant Frequency Breathing is uniquely powerful. When the heart rate is starting to speed up in perfect timing with the breath, it is beating fastest when there is the most oxygen available to distribute to the body. Your body can then get more oxygen and therefore more energy.

The other significant aspect of this practice which are relevant to Covid-19 is how this breathing method works on the nervous system. This breathing balances the two sides of the nervous system. While there are other yogic breathing exercise that have this effect, this method is the most accessible for our purposes. Most importantly, as it also switches on the Parasympathetic Nervous System, the healing response of the body initiates to reduce chronic inflammation. As we mentioned earlier, chronic inflammation is what makes the alveoli of your lungs fill up with fluid making it hard to transfer the oxygen.

Finally, when we breathe at this frequency and balance and nervous system, it reduces panic, anxiety, and depression. It helps to restore a sense of well-being and calmness that you will immediately feel.

As already mentioned, this is a very simple practice. All you do is count while inhaling and count again while you exhale. Being present in the moment is an added advantage. You can keep your eyes open or closed and as always, practice in the position that is most comfortable for you. With each exhalation, try to relax a little more. Imagine the tension leaving your body with the exhalation. Try not to pause between inhaling and exhaling. Imagine your breath moving in a circle.

This will be the longest part of each session and should be practiced for up to fifteen minutes, with a minimum of ten minutes to begin with.

11. Establishing a Recovery Practice

With these powerful, but simple breathing techniques, you now have the foundation of a practice that will aid you in your recovery from Covid-19 or what has been termed Long Covid. Most importantly this practice will speed up this recovery. Regular practice that lasts through time is important and giving yourself time to practice, twice a day, over the first fourteen days is crucial to aid in your recovery. Even just two weeks of this programme will have a long-term effect on your body. It is also helpful to try to do your practice at the same times each day and preferably in the same location. This repetition and familiarity will relax the body and mind and lead to a quicker recovery.

Each day for fourteen days, follow this programme:

1. Proper Deep Breathing – 5/10 Minutes

2. Kapalabhati – 5/10 Minutes
3. Bhramari -5/10 Minutes
4. Resonant Breathing – 10/15 Minutes

If you have any questions regarding this practice or any other methods which you may be interested in, please do not hesitate to reach out to me via email.

Dermot Ryan

Galway, IRELAND

December 2020

Practice and all is coming – B.K.S. Iyengar